Ketogenic Diet
For
Beginners

Learn the Secret to Eating Well, Losing Weight and Keeping It Off

Ron Kness

Sneak Peek

The story behind this book is my wife and I were looking for a healthy eating lifestyle change to lose the last few pounds we wanted to lose. After reading article after article of movie stars and other famous people raving about the Ketogenic diet, known as just Keto, we decided to learn as much as we could about it and try it. For those not familiar with its principles, it is low carb/high fat/high protein diet.

The science behind it is that the body converts carbohydrates into glucose and uses that for energy if carbs are available. And the excess carbs the body does not need are stored as bodyfat to be used during times where there is not a lot of food available. Unfortunately, that last part doesn't happen and consequently, we just keep getting fatter and fatter.

However, what is interesting is if there are not enough carbohydrates available, the body will convert fat into ketones and use that for energy. As a matter of fact, research has shown the body would prefer using ketones if it had the choice as it uses these more efficiently.

So, on the Keto diet, you restrict carbs, but not eliminate, and supply your body with fat and protein. If the body needs more ketones, then it taps the bodyfat sources to get more, which is where the weight loss comes in.

So far, after being on it about a month at the time of this writing, I lost my last 5 pounds and my wife her last six pounds. Because we typically do not eat a lot of things with sugar, which is a major source of carbohydrates – simple carbohydrates that quickly digest and spike blood sugar levels - it was an easy transition for us.

During my research, I found some people on the Keto diet were also doing intermittent fasting. That is they "fast" or don't eat, from about 6pm at night to 7am in the morning anyway so doing the 16:8 fast – fasting for 16 hours and eating during the remaining 8 hours. The Keto diet and intermittent fasting complement each other very well. While Keto is "what" and "how much" we eat, fasting is the "when" we eat. Combined, it is a one/two punch for not only losing weight but keeping it off for good.

If interested in fasting, I cover it and the Keto diet in my new upcoming book: ***Ketogenic Diet and Intermittent Fasting – The One/Two Punch for Lasting Weight Loss***.

With most other diets, you might lose weight in the short term, but as soon as you go off it, the weight comes right back on (and usually more). And because most diets are so restrictive, you can't stay on them forever. Eventually the craving for the foods you can't have while on that diet kick in and as you know from experience, the cravings win out every time.

But the Keto diet is different as you will see in this book. As a matter of fact, it does not seem like a diet at all but a healthy eating lifestyle that you could stay on for life if you choose to do so.

And as an incentive to try the Keto diet, I invite you to take advantage of my 14-day meal plan, including shopping lists and 75 recipes for dishes in the meal plan … it is free so why not opt to get it now!

If you are looking for a "diet" that doesn't seem like a diet at all, then I think you will find this one interesting, different and worth a try. The Keto diet worked for of us as it has for many that have tried it. What do you have to lose?

Read on to see what the Keto diet is about it can work for you ….

Contents

No part of this book may be reproduced, stored in a retrieval system, or transmitted in any form or by any means, electronic, mechanical, photocopying, recording, scanning, or otherwise, without the prior written permission of the publisher, except for the inclusion of brief quotations in a review.

This book is for **personal use only**.

Published by:

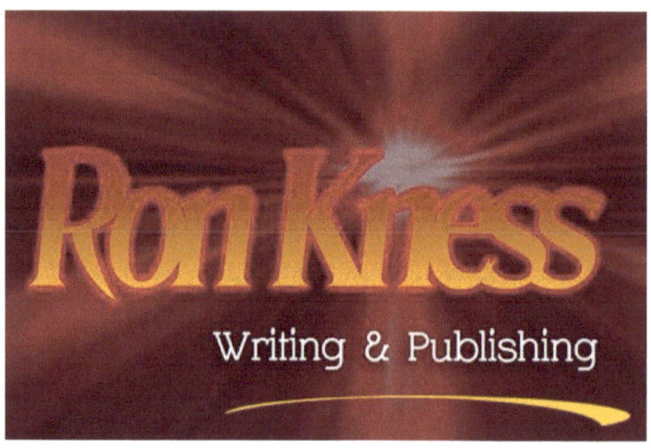

https://ronknesswriting.com

Ron Kness

San Tan Valley, AZ

United States of America

ISBN: 9781695384279

Disclaimer

This publication is for informational purposes only and is not intended as medical advice. Medical advice should always be obtained from a qualified medical professional for any health conditions or symptoms associated with them.

Every possible effort has been made in preparing and researching this material. We make no warranties with respect to the accuracy, applicability of its contents or any omissions.

See your healthcare professional before starting any diet, health or exercise program!

Introduction

Millions of people have made the switch to Keto successfully and with this book in your hands, you too can make the switch to a healthier eating lifestyle. If you want more energy, fast fat loss results and an overall improvement to your health and then the Keto lifestyle is exactly what you want. Another benefit my wife and I both experienced is less brain fog. We have more clarity and attentiveness since starting on this diet.

Part of being successful with the Keto diet is understanding how our bodies work and how specifically, dieting works.

Atkins, Weight Watchers, Slimming World, South Beach and more – the list of fad diets and lifestyle changes goes on and on, and it seems a new one is announced as being the next big celeb diet almost every week!

Unfortunately, a lot of these diets require severely limiting calorie intake, eating bland and boring food or even eating food that's not even solid as in some of the juicing and smoothie diets! There are numerous problems with all these diets, such as them not being nutritionally appropriate for long term use, being hard to stick to and almost all of them are not even worth your time because they simply don't work – and if they do in the short-term, none of them carry over into the long-term.

The only mainstream diets that show any real promise are diets like the Atkins diet – which to be fair has been around for a very long time… probably because it does work, it's just not particularly easy to follow and stick to – and people think of the Atkins diet as dated and old fashioned.

The background of the Atkins diet, however, is something you should pay attention to. Low-carb diets are the only ones that really seem to work and work fast – and not only that but they tend to work long-term as well.

Low-Carb Diets

Low-carb diets are one of the only diets that show improvements to health in the long term for conditions such as blood sugar problems, insulin levels and of course diabetes. This is because of the way your body processes the sugar in carbohydrates.

Carbohydrates are broken down by your body into glucose (the simplest form of sugar) and this then raises your blood sugar levels. Insulin in the body works to reduce this spike in blood sugar levels. These processes are part of how our bodies work. However, over the years, our bodies can end up needing to produce more and more insulin in order to reduce the blood sugar levels. This can quickly lead to prediabetes conditions because your body can end up insulin resistant. In other words, your body no longer reacts to the same amount of insulin that it once did.

Insulin resistance, pre-diabetes, metabolic syndrome and Type 2 diabetes are genuine problems that people are facing every day because of high sugar in their diets. Our diets are increasingly high in carbs and sugar and convenience, fast and processed foods are really compounding the problem.

According to recent statistics by the American Diabetes Association, more than 1 in 3 adults in the USA have prediabetes and nearly 1 in 10 Americans have Type 2 diabetes. These numbers aren't limited to the U.S. either. Parts of Europe and the rest of the developed world are seeing similar rises and figures when looking at diabetes.

Diet Changes Have Caused Obesity

Obesity and diet have a huge role to play in these figures. Since the 1980s, obesity has risen across the world and in the U.S. alone, obesity has risen from just 15 percent in the 80s, to over 35 percent in the present day.

There is blatant evidence that shows these figures are the direct results of our changing diet (and not for the better) over the decades. The first ever dietary guide was released in the 80s and their recommendations were to reduce fats, oils and sweets – makes sense.

However, they also recommended that carbohydrates were among the foods that were to take up a large portion of your plate for each meal.

This advice is even used today. The food pyramid was released after the above recommendations and the largest section of this pyramid is for carbohydrates. The recommendation of 6-11 portions per day is absurd. They also recommend eating 2-4 portions of fruit which is also high in sugars – albeit natural sugar fructose, but still sugar.

Even decades later, these guidelines are what promote the high carb lifestyle that we all lead today and what continues to make us fatter. It's not that it's super unhealthy – especially if you're eating vegetables as well – it's just that high sugar diets are generally frowned upon today.

So, why do high sugar foods, such as carbohydrates and fruit, take such prominence on a food pyramid and recommended daily intake chart?

Trust Your Body To Do Its Thing

Your body does need glucose, but did you know that your body is actually quite capable of producing glucose through a process called gluconeogenesis. The liver can convert glycerol (which is derived from fats in your diet) into glucose. This essentially means that you don't NEED carbohydrates and sugary fruits to fulfil your body's glucose needs.

It's not just eating carbs that's causing problems though. You have probably been told that eating a high fat diet – particularly saturated fats are bad for you and cause heart disease and other health problems.

Now, we are finding out this information is very out of date and simply not true.

In the past decade, dozens of studies have disproven these facts. There have been a lot of studies that have shown there is no link between a high saturated fat diet and heart disease. There were also studies conducted with over 900,000 subjects from almost 100 different data sets and these studies showed almost the same conclusions – there is no long-term or short-term risk to eating saturated fats in your diet.

Fats are very good for our bodies and are essential to our health. That's why you hear people talking about essential fatty acids and "good fats". The fact is, most fats are actually good for you and the scare mongering that has gone on about certain types of fat has just gone too far.

Ketones, Ketosis and Ketogenic Diets

Fat is the most efficient form of energy and your body processes fat in an extremely efficient and effective way. When you change your diet to a high fat and high protein diet, while reducing your carb intake, your body actually uses this fat and protein (as well as the stored fat in your body) and converts it into what we call "ketones".

This whole process is called ketosis and ketones are one of the best sources of energy your body can use. The ketogenic diet is very good for you and can give you such a huge boost in energy levels that you will wonder why on earth the so-called experts were recommending you eat carbohydrates at all! Note, on the Keto diet you can still have up to 50 grams of carbs per day and still stay in ketosis.

Of course, this makes things very interesting. It means you must rethink your whole idea of dieting. What you have been taught in the past is essentially wrong. We have been fed this misinformation for so long that it took my wife and I a while to get past this and eat a low carb/ high fat/high protein Keto diet.

This book is here to teach you the essentials of the Keto diet so you learn how to do it right and to ensure you succeed with the Ketogenic diet.

What is the Keto Diet?

Want a diet that encourages bacon and eggs for breakfast? Then the Keto diet is exactly what you're looking for. In general, the Keto diet is about eating fresh produce and high protein meats, oils and fat, fish and vegetables and cutting out processed and high carb foods.

Because of the way your body processes these foods, it's actually a very easy diet to stick to (once through the initial stages).

It's a diet you can sustain for the long term and it isn't a fad or something that you can't stick to for the rest of your life. Unlike most other diets, we did not experience any food cravings.

Aside from the obvious benefits of weight loss, you will also find that the Keto diet will reduce your chances of things like diabetes, heart disease and even stroke, Alzheimer's, epilepsy and many more health conditions. As mentioned earlier, we experience less brain fog. Actually, the Keto diet was first developed to help people with epilepsy and later discovered it was good at reducing the risk of other diseases and conditions.

Due to the higher fat content of a Keto diet, you will find that you'll stay satiated longer and that your energy levels will improve – and last throughout the day. This is because of how our bodies process fats compared with carbohydrates for energy.

When you eat carbohydrates, your body produces blood glucose, and between this and the insulin response, can cause ups and downs in your blood sugar levels. This is part of what leads to diabetes. Ups and downs in blood sugars and your bodies constant need to produce insulin can result in insulin resistance which is what causes Type 2 diabetes. Or your adrenal glands must produce so much insulin that over time, they can't keep up and eventually wear out and fail.

In general, because of how our bodies process fat, you will feel fuller for longer and therefore overall eat fewer calories – aiding your weight loss even further and improving your overall health.

So, Why Go Keto?

I think we've made it pretty clear from the above information that there are many benefits to going Keto. However, let's look at this properly and really nail down the true reasons to change your diet to a Ketogenic one.

When you start a Ketogenic diet, you will be eating a higher fat diet than you're probably used to (or thought was ok!). Don't worry.

Your body becomes very efficient at burning fat for fuel and this in turn makes your body a more efficient energy machine.

Fat has almost double the calorie content of carbohydrates (9 for fat verses 4 for carbohydrates) and so you need to eat a lot less food to satisfy your body's needs. This means you eat less in general and what you do eat is processed properly and efficiently by your body.

As mentioned before, when you eat a high carbohydrate diet, your body will experience highs and lows in blood sugar. These spikes and dips in energy can really affect how you feel, i.e. "sugar crashes".

When your body uses fat for fuel instead, you won't experience these dips and therefore are likely to feel much more energised and far more productive throughout the day.

Obviously, the above benefits are noticeable shortly after starting the Keto diet and will be beneficial almost straight away. There are longer term benefits as well and these include things like more weight loss (specifically body fat as opposed to muscle mass and water), reduction in blood sugar levels (in turn reducing the risks of diabetes and other illnesses), reduction in triglyceride levels, blood pressure reductions, improved levels of cholesterols (increase in good, reduction in bad) and even improved brain function when it comes to things like concentration and productivity. I already mentioned that both my wife and I experience less brain fog and feel more alert!

Starting A Ketogenic Diet

In simple terms, when you eat a "normal" diet, which consists of high carbohydrate levels, your body uses primarily blood glucose for its energy. This means after each meal your body uses this source of energy to keep it going – unfortunately, this state promotes storage of body fat and blocks the release of fat from your stores.

When you eat a Ketogenic diet this process changes. If your primary source of energy comes from high fat and low carb diet, your body goes into a state called ketosis. This state promotes fat burning – including your fat stores. This is why you lose weight quickly and because your body has a constant flow of fat content (fat is slower to digest than carbs, so the ups and downs of your blood sugar levels are far fewer) from food and from your fat stores, you will find your energy levels are more consistent.

In other words, you don't get the energy crashes like you do when eating a diet high in carbohydrates. You have a good supply of bodyfat available that the body can convert to energy as it sees fit. With carbs, the body must wait until to you eat more carbs before it can convert it to energy.

Becoming Keto-Adapted

This is a term used to describe the state you want your body to be in when fully on the Keto diet. Basically, when you first start the Keto diet, your body will require some time to adapt. This process can take anywhere from 4 to 8 weeks and while for some that can seem like a long time, in the grand scheme of things, it really isn't.

Becoming Keto-adapted is about getting to a stage where the glucose in your muscles and liver reduce to a point where you carry less water weight, your muscle endurance increases, and your overall energy levels are higher. Before you start the Keto diet, your body will be in a different state of processing glucose and sugars, etc. so it can take time for your body to adjust to this new process of creating energy.

In fact, making sure that you get to the Keto-adapted stage is, and should be, your primary goal. Once you reach this stage, you can actually rely on your body and ketosis to a greater extent. For example, when fully Keto-adapted, you can eat up to 50 grams of carbs a day and still remain in ketosis. For me, I like to use some of my carb grams to have real cream in my coffee – one little pleasure I refuse to give up, and it is legal on the Keto diet as long as I stay to 50 grams for day or less. Also, if you mess up after you've become Keto-adapted, your body will return to a Ketosis state much quicker than it would have done before.

Starting A Ketogenic Diet with Diabetes

Obviously, if you have a condition like diabetes, or any condition that is diet dependent or sensitive, you will need to consult your doctor first before changing your eating habits significantly. However, a Ketogenic diet has been proven to be very helpful for those with diabetes – both Type 1 and 2.

With Type 1 diabetes, it can help control blood sugar levels, but you should make sure you speak with your doctor to ensure your medications are at the right levels for a new diet. You may even have to consider a trial run with medical supervision to begin with. And if you are diabetic, you also need to be aware of a condition called ketoacidosis - a toxic metabolic state that happens when your body can't regulate the ketone production. If left unchecked, it can be fatal; non-diabetics have nothing to worry about. To avoid this, you will probably need to eat over 50 grams of carbohydrates every day – but please consult your doctor for specific advice.

Because Type 2 diabetes is a lifestyle disease, changing your lifestyle over to the Keto diet can reduce and reverse the condition altogether. Imagine life again without having to take insulin!

Getting The Keto Diet Right

As with any diet, there are things you actually need to make sure you're doing and the most important one is that you are balancing the diet nutritionally. You need to make sure that you are getting the right proteins and fats into your diet and that you aren't missing any essential nutrients.

To do this, you will need to learn about the ratios involved and about macronutrients. Macronutrients is a term used to describe when parts of foods provide energy per gram consumed. In other words, it's about what you eat and how much energy it gives you – more commonly referred to as how many calories are in the food!

The calorie breakdown of the three macronutrients …

- Fat contains about 9 calories per gram
- Protein contains about 4 calories per gram
- Carbohydrates provide about 4 calories per gram

You will need to work on your diet by changing ratios so that your diet is about 65-75% fat, 20-25% protein and only 5% from carbohydrates.

Tracking the Keto diet

There are online trackers you can use to make sure you are hitting your nutritional and keto goals. Generally, you don't need to stick to a super strict set of numbers to actually see results. This is one of the many reasons that Keto diets are so popular. Actually, tracking the Keto diet and your intake of calories (in the right ratios) is simple.

Below is an example of a 2,000 calorie per day guide to show you the levels in percentages and number of grams of food you should be eating for each macronutrient …

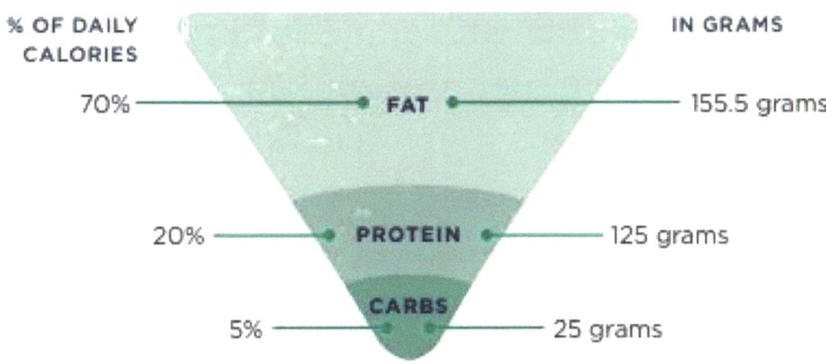

Obviously, 2,000 calories per day is just an example. You will have your own goals and your own needs calorie-wise. You will need to take a few things into account before you set your goals.

Start by figuring out how many calories you need each day just to survive. This is called your Resting Metabolic Rate. Next add in your activity factor based on how much you exercise and how active you are throughout the day. This figure is your Active Metabolic Rate and is the number of calories you need each day to maintain your current weight.

Of course, if you want to lose weight, then your calories that you burn must be more than the calories you eat – generally around 500 per day more. This will give you a weight loss of around 1 to 2 pounds per week which is considered a safe loss-rate.

Like any diet, your goals and targets will likely be based on your current situation. For example, do you have a lot of weight to lose? What is your current lean body weight? What are your activity levels? Are you going to be exercising a lot?

Most importantly, your overall goals will come into play. Do you want to lose weight? Maintain weight? Gain muscle? Things like this will decide how much you will need calorie-wise each day. You can use online calculators to figure all this out down to the specific numbers.

What is Keto Flu?

This is a term used to describe the first weeks of the Keto diet. It's unfortunate for some people, but with a huge lifestyle change like going Keto, there are side effects, but they are temporary. Many people, like my wife and I for example did not have any Keto flu symptoms. These side effects are just the process of your body changing the way it deals with your intake and it is mainly the result of your body flushing toxins and other things out of your system. If you are addicted to sugar and have eaten a lot of it each day, you may experience Keto flu symptoms when you reduce the amount each day.

When you start a Keto diet, it is important that you drink a lot of water. Your body will start flushing the sodium stores in your body – these sodium stores are what builds up when we eat a highly processed diet. When you switch to Keto you will be eating more wholesome and natural foods. This will kick start your body into flushing excess sodium. You body will also notice a reduction in carbohydrates and therefore insulin production – this will also promote your kidneys to release excess stored sodium.

Because of all this, your body will be excreting a lot more water than usual, and you may notice you'll be going to the toilet a lot more than usual. Therefore, water intake is important – you need to keep hydrated and drinking lots of water will improve your body's ability to flush these things out and speed up the process.

The reason you feel rough with symptoms such as headaches, fatigue and potentially irritability and nausea is because your body will be low on electrolytes during this phase. It's very important to remember that the "Keto flu" is just a nickname for flu-like symptoms and it's not an actual illness.

Unfortunately, a lot of people who start the Keto diet will experience these symptoms and then go straight back to eating carbs. It's important to fight through this phase and get to the other side. The other side is where all the benefits are.

There are ways to reduce the symptoms of Keto flu and it's important to remember that it only lasts a few days while your body adjusts.

Easing Symptoms of Keto Flu

The causes of "Keto flu" are generally to do with low sodium while your body flushes out stored sodium from the processed foods you used to eat. However, there are ways to increase your sodium intake, therefore reducing the symptoms of Keto flu, without eating processed foods.

The obvious way is to add salt to all your meals, drink soup and broth type meals and things like bacon and pickles are good.

You can also replace other electrolytes such as potassium, magnesium and calcium. Even phosphorus and chloride can be replaced by eating the right foods.

Here's a little chart which should help you reduce the symptoms of Keto flu.

ELECTROLYTE	FOODS CONTAINING ELECTROLYTE
POTASSIUM	Avocados, nuts, dark leafy greens such as spinach and kale, salmon, plain yogurt, mushrooms
MAGNESIUM	Nuts, dark chocolate, artichokes, spinach, fish
CALCIUM	Cheeses, leafy greens, broccoli, seafood, almonds
PHOSPHORUS	Meats, cheeses, nuts, seeds, dark chocolate
CHLORIDE	Most vegetables, olives, salt, seaweed

Getting Support from Family & Friends

To get yourself off to the best start, it's a good idea to ensure you let your family and friends know how serious you are about following the Keto diet. They will need to know what foods you want to avoid and how they can cater to you in social situations without it being a big deal.

You will find some friends and family are initially a little sceptical or perhaps not supportive, but this will pass. Stick to your guns and make sure you think of your long-term goals and stay focused. Once they see how much weight you have lost on the Keto diet, they may join you!

If you are struggling to get support from your direct family and friends, then you can always join support forums and places like Reddit where you will find like minded people and other Keto goers who are in the same position as you.

Testing For Ketosis

Now that you've made the initial steps to going Keto, you will want to make sure that you are actually in ketosis and it can be tricky to tell. However, there are ways to test your state of ketosis.

It's a great motivator to see that you are in ketosis and to understand that you have done the right things. This makes it easier to stick to the diet because you feel a sense of pride in that you did the right things and eating the right foods.

One of the most common and easy ways to test for ketosis is by noticing a change in your breath. Sounds odd doesn't it? Basically, when you enter ketosis your body excretes acetone in your urine and breath. It's a fruity smell/taste and some people even describe it as metallic – but some people may not notice it at all.

The most accurate way of testing for ketosis is by using urine test strips. You can buy these at most pharmacies or online and they usually come in bulk packs. Your best bet is to use the sticks a few hours after you've woken up each day – first morning urine isn't the best as dehydration can give a false positive.

You can even opt for a blood test if you want to be absolutely sure but unless you're doing this for certain medical reasons – like dealing with diabetes – then it's not really necessary to go that far.

As you get further into the diet, you will find that you don't need to test as often. Once you know how to follow the diet and you've tested positive for ketosis, you'll know what to do to keep yourself there.

Go Keto In Just 5 Steps

Now that you know the science behind the Keto diet and how it actually works, now it's time to put it all into practice. The next section covers how to go Keto in just five simple steps. This is an easy step-by-step guide to get you started on the Keto diet.

Step 1: Clean Out Your Kitchen

First things first, you can't go Keto if your whole house is full of carbohydrates and tempting sugary foods, unless you have terrific will power, which you probably don't or you would not be looking at the Keto diet to lose weight. It's really important to start this diet well prepared and that means making sure that you don't have any temptations at home.

This can be difficult if you don't live alone. Try and explain to your housemates or family that you are going Keto and that any tempting snacks or foods will need to perhaps be kept in different locations.

Things to get rid of

Starches & Grains

Things like cereals, rice, pasta, potatoes, corn, oats, quinoa, flour, bread, bagels, rolls, wraps and croissants all must go.

Sugary Foods & Drinks

Get rid of all drinks like fruit juices, milk, desserts, pastries, milk chocolate and candy.

Legumes

Beans, peas and lentils are a no go. They are super high in carbs. Beans alone contain about three times the amount of carbs you want to consume.

Processed Polyunsaturated Fats and Oils

Get rid of all vegetable oils and seed oils, such as sunflower, grapeseed and corn oil. Margarine and trans fats are a big no-no as well. Anything that says "hydrogenated" or "partially hydrogenated" is what you want to avoid.

Fruits

Fruits that are high in carbs include things like bananas, dates, grapes, mangos and apples. Dried fruits like raisins are also not allowed.

It may feel like you've just emptied your entire kitchen! To be honest, it will basically be exactly that. You will probably notice that a lot of high carb food and high sugar food tends to be food that is kept in your cupboards. Fresh food and food that's healthy and Keto friendly will mostly be kept in your fridge – with a few exceptions like healthy oils.

Step 2: Go Shopping

This part is where you'll refill your kitchen with everything Keto friendly that you're going to eat.

Here is a list of things you can stock your kitchen with that can be essentially called "basics". You can eat and drink all these things.

- Water, coffee and tea
- Spices and herbs
- Sweeteners including things like stevia and erythritol
- Lemon and lime juice
- Low carb condiments such as mayonnaise, mustard and pesto
- Broths (things like chicken and beef)
- Pickled foods like pickles, kimchi and sauerkraut
- Nuts and seeds such as macadamia nuts, pecans, almonds, walnuts, hazelnuts, pine nuts, chia seeds and pumpkin seeds

Meat

All meats such as pork, chicken, lamb, beef and turkey, etc. are options. You can buy all these, and you don't have to worry about the fat and skin – eat it all. You should opt for organic if you can afford it but either way it's fine.

Fish

All fish is fine too – but try to avoid farmed fish if you can. Sustainable wild-caught is always better.

Other proteins

Eggs are a staple in the Keto diet, and you'll find them a huge part of your new diet. Get free-range or organic or both if you can.

Vegetables

You want to focus on non-starchy vegetables, such as broccoli, mushrooms, cucumbers, lettuce, onions, peppers, tomatoes, garlic, asparagus, brussels sprouts, zucchini, eggplant, olives and cauliflower.

You will need to avoid literally all potatoes, yams, sweet potatoes, corn and things like beans, lentils and peas.

Fruits

Berries such as strawberries, raspberries, blackberries and blueberries are all ok in small amounts each day. Lemons and limes are ideal for flavouring meals and you can eat plenty of avocado which is high in good fat and low in carbs.

Most other fruit is very high in carbs and therefore it's safest to avoid.

Dairy

If you eat dairy in your diet, then always opt for the full-fat version. Butter, sour cream, heavy cream, cheese and cream cheese – all fine if they're the full-fat versions. You should avoid things like milk, skimmed milk and sweetened yoghurts. They are too high in sugar. Don't buy anything that says it's flavoured, low-fat or fat-free.

Fats & Oils

There are oils you can use that are Keto-friendly. Avocado, olive oil, and of course butter, are all fine. Bacon fat is great for cooking too. A little tip – avocado oil is really great for cooking because it has a really high burn temperature which basically means it doesn't smoke much and so are ideal in frying pans and for searing meat. Don't buy any oils that say "blend" as they usually use a lot of unhealthy oils to bulk them up.

Below is a handy chart which will show you some healthy Keto-friendly alternatives to your usual purchases. This might make shopping a little bit easier!

NOT SO FRIENDLY	NET CARBS	QUANTITY	KETO-FRIENDLY ALTERNATIVE	NET CARBS
Milk	13 grams	1 cup	Unsweetened almond milk	0 grams
Pasta	41 grams	1 cup	Zucchini noodles	3 grams
Wraps or tortillas	18 grams	1 medium	Low-carb tortillas	6 grams
Sugar	25 grams	2 tablespoons	Stevia or erythritol	0 grams
Rice	44 grams	1 cup	Shirataki rice	0 grams
Mashed potatoes	22 grams	½ cup	Mashed cauliflower	4 grams
Bread crumbs	36 grams	½ cup	Almond flour	6 grams
Soda	39 grams	12 ounces	Water, tea, or coffee	0 grams
French fries	44 grams	4 ounces	Zucchini fries	3 grams
Potato chips	46 grams	3½ ounces	Mixed nuts	14 grams

If you want to kick-start your Keto diet, be sure to get my 14-Day Eating Plan complete with shopping list for the dishes in the plan and the recipes for making the dishes. It is free; just click here!

Step 3: Setting Up Your Kitchen

You should probably get used to the idea of having to cook all your meals now. Yes, for some this can be a bit of a pain but once you get the hang of it it's fun – and part of the joys of living Keto.

Of course, we all lead busy lives and with families, full time jobs and other commitments, we all want things that are going to help speed things up. These tips are designed to ensure your kitchen is set up to make things simple and easy while you're cooking your delicious Keto meals.

Kitchen Scales

Measuring can be a bit of a chore, but with Ketogenic diets, it's important to get your measurements right. Kitchen scales aren't expensive, and you can easily weigh each piece of food or liquid you cook or use to cook, and this makes tracking things a whole lot easier. You can even pair this with apps on your phone to ensure you know the calories as well.

Electric Hand Mixer

This kind of depends on what you eat, but if you've ever had to hand whisk something for a recipe, you'll understand why we're suggesting an electric hand mixer. It's just easier!

Spiralizer

These are great and can make meals so much more enjoyable and exciting. You can use them to make things like noodles with vegetables. We spiralize zucchini and use it as a replacement for spaghetti or as a vegetable.

A Food Processor

One step further than the hand mixer, a food processor will give you so many options when making meals. You can blend foods and get really creative with your recipes. Tough vegetables like cauliflowers aren't going to blend well in a simple smoothie maker or blender so a food processor is a must.

Cast Iron Pans

These are great! You can use them on both the top and in the oven, which makes them versatile for cooking. They also aren't chemically treated which means you don't need to worry about non-stick stuff coming off into your food! You'll also find they last a lot longer and don't rust, if taken care of properly – so they're a good investment regardless of your diet!

Step 4: Following Meal Plans

One of the things that will greatly increase your chances of success early in the Keto diet will be following meal plans.

Having direction and plans make following this diet much easier in the beginning. Plus knowing what's coming next and not having to wait around thinking on the spot of what to eat can be a life saver. You're much less likely to call for your favorite takeout if you already have a meal plan and the food in your kitchen ready to go. You only really need to use meal plans for a few weeks until you're settled. Once you've got the hang of things, it'll be easier to follow ad-hoc. Be sure to download the bonus book I have for you. It has a 14-day meal plan, shopping list for the dishes in the plan and 75 recipes on how to prepare the dishes in the plan. This will get you started on the right track. Click here to get it free!

You should also consider customising meal plans and making sure that they are what you want to eat ahead of time. There's no point in following meal plans where some of the foods aren't really your cup of tea – remember, there are so many options when following Keto that you shouldn't really find yourself very restricted. And if you do a search for Keto dishes online, you will be flooded with options – most downloadable for free!

You don't have to stick strictly to home cooked meals. There are options you can look at when shopping if you want easy "ready-meals". However, you will be very limited when trying to find pre-packaged meals that aren't processed, full of sugar and high in carbs. If you do look then you need to know what you're looking for. Look at the labels and make sure that you understand what's in the foods – most of the best foods contain hardly any ingredients – when in doubt, just buy the products with the fewest ingredients and make sure to avoid sugary, carb-laden meals.

Step 5: Exercising on Keto

Exercise isn't completely necessary to lose weight while on the Keto diet. However, if you're looking at overall health, then you will want to increase your activity levels. This should be easier than you may think given that your overall energy levels are going to increase while on the diet – you may find yourself doing more without really trying.

If you want to increase your exercise, then it's a good idea to start gradually – especially if you are currently quite sedate. If you live a sedentary lifestyle, then you will find it difficult to just jump into a major exercise regime. Luckily, with the Keto diet, you will be motivated by the progress you make before you even start lifting weights or doing cardio-type!

Cardio is important for heart health and overall fitness and building your muscles will help you burn more fat both now and over the long-term. Why? Because it takes more calories to maintain muscle then it does fat, so as your bodyfat levels go down and your muscle mass goes up, you will naturally burn more calories than before. In other words, your Resting Metabolic Rate will be higher than before. This means a combination of cardio exercise and strength training is the best way to go about it.

Take your time and don't feel you need to do it all at once. Making sure you are just doing a little extra every day is the ideal way to approach this.

Conclusion

This guide has shown you all the benefits of a Keto diet, including all the steps you need to take to get started. We covered the scientific side of things so that you really understand the Keto diet and how it all works. We then looked at how it can help you and the benefits to your overall health.

If you are looking to start a Keto diet, then good luck and we hope this guide has helped you to understand how it all works and how best to approach it!

Now the rest is up to you. Get started!

Ketogenic Cheat Sheet

FOOD	SERVING SIZE	CARBS (GRAMS)	CALORIES
POTATO	1 large, baked, plain	56 grams	283
RICE	1 cup, white or brown	50 grams	223
OATMEAL	1 cup, dry	49 grams	339
PINTO BEANS (COOKED)	1 cup	45 grams	245
BAGEL	1 whole	44 grams	245
YOGHURT	1 cup, fruit-flavored, low-fat	42 grams	225
CORN (COOKED)	1 cup	41 grams	177
SPAGHETTI	1 cup	40 grams	221
PIZZA	1 slice, cheese	39 grams	290
APPLE JUICE	1 cup	28 grams	113
SWEET POTATO	1 large	28 grams	118
ORANGE JUICE	1 cup	26 grams	112
ENGLISH MUFFIN	1 whole	25 grams	130
WAFFLE	1 (7-inch diameter)	25 grams	218
BANANA	1 medium	24 grams	105
APPLE	1 medium	21 grams	81

CEREAL, READY TO EAT	1 cup	18 grams	103
PANCAKE	1 (5-inch diameter)	15 grams	90
MILK	1 cup	12 grams	103
BREAD	1 slice, white	12 grams	66
GREEN PEAS	½ a cup	12 grams	63
STRAWBERRIES	1 cup	11 grams	45
CUCUMBER	1 (8-inch length)	9 grams	47
YELLOW ONION	1 medium	8 grams	44
BROCCOLI	1 stalk	6 grams	51
ZUCCHINI	1 medium	4 grams	33
CARROT	1 medium	4 grams	25
TOMATO	1 medium	3 grams	22
WHITE MUSHROOMS	1 cup	2 grams	15
EGG	1 large	0.6 grams	78
SPINACH	1 cup	0.4 grams	7

14-Day Meal Plan, Shopping List and Recipes

As mentioned, several times throughout this book I have a 14-Day Meal Plan available for download. Not only does it have options to eat for breakfast, lunch and dinner, but also the shopping lists for the dishes in the plan and the 75 recipes for making the dishes in the plan. It is a quick guide to get you up and running on the Keto diet. Just click here to download it.

About the Author

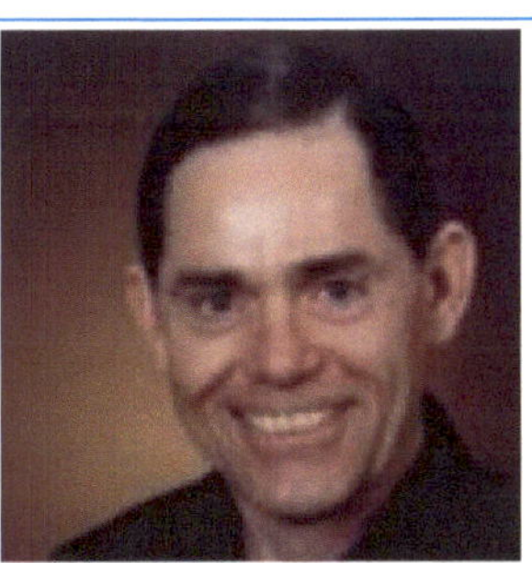

I have published numerous books on Amazon (both for Kindle and in paperback), along with other publishing platforms.

While most of my books are on health and fitness in general, I also write on baby boomer and older citizen health issues and have a recent interest in creating and printing journals/ planners and other printable products.

Besides my own writing, I also ghostwrite ebooks, books, reports, articles, blogs and do Kindle conversions for clients on a variety of topics.

Go to my website at http://ronknesswriting.com for more information or to submit a quote. For a complete list of my books, go to https://www.amazon.com/Ron-Kness/e/B0072M6PYO.

Today my wife and I are retired from our careers and live in San Tan Valley, AZ. I now write as a retirement business where you'll find me happily sitting in my office typing away on my laptop as I work on my next book or ghostwriting project . . . that is if we are not traveling on a cruise ship - our new-found mode of travel.